1

A Man's Guide to the Female Workplace

By: *Chad Dyer*

Preface:

Hi my name is Chad. I'm going to jump right in and say that I'm not a writer, nor am I psychologist. I'm just a man who's worked in healthcare for 26 years. I started out at my local nursing home as an orderly and later completed the training for a C.N.A. position. I've worked in numerous nursing homes, psychiatric units, and hospitals. I went on to become a P.C.T., which is a cross between an L.P.N. and a C.N.A. During this time I worked very closely with R.N.s. The job required everything from daily care and hygiene, foley catheters, wound care, tube feedings, to charting and data entry. The P.C.T. positions were later replaced. I looked into other positions available and

learned I could transfer to the lab as a phlebotomist /
dispatcher. This involves travel in the hospital from
patient to patient, and obtaining blood samples for
processing in the lab. At other times, it requires
receiving orders from the entire hospital and
dispatching other phlebotomists out. This brings us to
now- and why I am writing this book.

Through the years I've found it difficult, yes
sometimes exhausting; mentally, physically,
spiritually, and emotionally, to work with the opposite
sex. Some examples that come to mind are: only being
able to use certain, (unisex) bathrooms, being blamed
for other men's mistakes - i .e. "Why do men do this or
that? Why is my boyfriend/husband a jerk?" Or being
used for my stature and physical strength when being

assigned the heaviest workload, as well as being sexually harassed. There's much more, but I'd need a whole book for that amount of venting. This book is only designed to be a guide. It includes some rules that I've learned along the way to keep me safe, and I think that other men could benefit from these rules also.

Since this is intended as a general guide, it's not going to be long and drawn out. I'm going to try to keep it short and to the point.

And now onto the guide…

Chapter One:

Do Not Engage Subjects to Never Speak On

From the title of this chapter, you can tell I'm a huge Star Trek fan, and just like Captain Picard says *engage* or *do not engage*, every conversation or anything you want to say while in the workplace needs to be under the same scrutiny. For example, some of the subjects that will come from your coworkers, could be how heavy their "flow" is that month, which Doctor is going to impregnate them, or one of your coworkers may even come up to you and say "hey I put myself on sugarbabies.com gonna flirt with some men and get them to pay my bills". Be aware that nothing is off the table when it comes to these conversations, so you need to be ready for anything.

RULE ONE: *Never talk about anything sexual.*

We all talk about sex, but some women may talk about it in such detail, you might as well have been in the room with them. So, if someone starts to talk about anything sexual, do yourself a favor and say I don't think this is appropriate for work, and dismiss yourself by saying there is something you have to do. You could say you need to go to the bathroom, but seriously - just walk away. When it comes to the subject of sex while at work, the rule is simple: don't talk about it, don't joke about it, don't mention it, because really man, sex has no place in the workplace.

Which brings me to…

RULE TWO: *Never bring up workplace crushes.*

One of these days a coworker will be talking about: *who they think is hot, who turns them on,* or *who is fire.* You may guess what's next, yes - they will inevitability turn to you and ask who you like or who turns you on? This can only go one of two ways. First scenario, you tell them. You can trust and believe that this information will find its way to that person, and things will get super awkward. I mean seriously, you guys have to work together and she may not feel the same, or she may have a boyfriend/husband, or she may be gay. She may even start making fun of you.

In the second scenario, she may like you and the two of you go on a date. In the beginning, it's awesome, because you guys hit it off, you always have something to talk about, laugh about and you can vent to one another. You may even carpool together. Soon your female coworkers are showing you all sorts of attention and I tell you man, it's like glory days back in high school. There's one problem with this scenario, you're not in high school. You are in the workplace, because you are an adult with bills, and there is no summer break. So, eventually you guys break up or grow apart. When it happened to me, she started to spread rumors and everyone thought I was a jerk. Now that may not happen to you, but everyone knows when a breakup happens it's as unpredictable as a star exploding.

RULE THREE: *Never talk about men's issues.*

Trust me, you will overhear women talking

about all the issues they go through. This may include: *how their dad treated them, how the world treats them, hormones, emotions, periods, weight, shaving, hair care, pregnancy, the wage gap, feminism,* etc. I have to tell ya, they do go through a lot. However, so do men. Unfortunately, in the workplace it has been my experience that most women do not care about men's issues .

It is my personal belief that most women are smarter than most men, but they use their intellect in the wrong way. So, if you were to talk to a woman about men's issues, there is the risk they may take your words, twist them, and throw them back in your face. This has happened to me too many times. For example, if a woman confronts you about women's issues, with that anger and fire in their eyes, there is only one counter response that will work. It goes like this: *stand your ground, look them in the eye, listen,* and after they're done talking, say "I'm so sorry you have to go through that. The world is so hard on us all, good luck and God bless you."

RULE FOUR: *How to comment on a woman's looks.*

If you're like me and work in a hospital, you may be surrounded by a lot of attractive women. Like many men, there's always going to be that teenage kid in the back of your mind wanting to blurt out "Wow you're pretty!" or "Damn you're hot!" The fact is, you have to be a man and take that kid, find a closet in your mind to throw him in and lock the door.

Now, there are some things that I've found you can comment on without being punched in the face. First their hair. If you see a woman that's done something different with her hair and you like it, providing you know them well, you could say, "Hey I like what you've done with your hair it looks nice". Perhaps she has painted her nails. You could say, "Nice color, it matches what you're wearing". In addition, if she has a nice pair of shoes, a nice jacket, or another clothing item, you could give her a compliment on that clothing item.

Be advised, you do not want to make comments like, "Hey nice jeans, love how they make your butt look," or, "Nice heels, like how they complement your legs." One last thing. For some reason, and I don't know what that reason is, you can compliment hair, nails, and clothing items, but if a woman has been working out and she's looking real good, you can never ever say how good she looks. Whether positive or negative, commenting on a woman's body is off limits.

RULE FIVE: *Just remember etiquette.*

As with any job, or any public place, just like your parents said, *be on your best behavior*. In other words, try to refrain from talking politics, religion, and always preface an answer with "in my opinion", not as facts.

Chapter Two:

Hands Off and Safety Zones

This may be one of my shortest chapters, because I hope everyone knows to not touch a woman without her consent. This should just be a refresher. (If you don't know that simple truth, seriously, please stop reading this guide. Go talk with and listen to your mother.) I can usually make it through the whole shift without touching anyone, with the exception of my patients, but there are a few cases where you'll have to, so here's my advice. When saying hi for the first time, or the hundreth, a hello should be good enough. If you do anything more, it should just be a handshake.

If, however, you've worked with them long enough, and have become workplace friends, maybe a fist bump. If you've known them a long time and you're very good workplace friends, there's one other place that's safe and (I emphasize), only in certain situations. That would be a pat on the back, to say they did a great job on something, or they're going through a hard time. When I say the back, I'm actually talking about the shoulder blades not the center of the back and not the outside of the shoulder. Now sometimes a woman will want to hug. Again, be sure you know the woman well as a workplace friend, and make sure you *never* initiate the hug, and only hug a woman if she is coming in to hug you first .

Chapter Three:

Workplace Socializing, and How it Works...at

Work

Now this is going to be another short chapter, because

I've never been a social butterfly. For me to get invited

anywhere, whether workplace or personal, is rare. So,

take that into consideration when reading this chapter.

As far as I have observed, men and women approach

work with different perspectives. For example: Not all

men, but men like myself, could go to work and never

really socialize with anyone. At least no one outside of

"need to know information". However, a lot of women

need more. They forge friendships and even hang out

apart from work. I also realize that not all men take

the, "need to know," approach. So, I offer some

suggestions based on my experiences working with women. My suggestion is simple: *change it up a bit, be polite* and *show respect*. I call this approach *care and share*. First, ask them about their family, where they're from, and their interests. This shows that you "care". Then, you "share" with them about your interests, your family and your family's pets, etc.

Now, my next point may appear to be stating the obvious. What you do not want to do is participate in gossip...with anyone. I've found the best thing that works is just to be honest. For example, I have said "I'm sorry I'm not comfortable talking about (insert name) when they are not around." If you are good at redirecting a conversation, now would be a good time to do that. Even standing in the same area listening to the gossip could be received as you agreeing with them about whatever is being gossiped about. That's going to be crazy if you later have someone in your face asking if you were talking about them. Backpedaling is hard... Trust me, it's not going to end well.

Some additional suggestions for consideration are: *think about character development*. What do I mean by this? After you've worked together in the same workplace a month or so, you might begin to insert a little of yourself into the conversation, becoming personable. What does this look like? Things to consider sharing might be: *hobbies*, *pets*, *music*, *foods you like*, and if you are comfortable with the topic of spouse or partner, this could be a *positive* to share also. In my workplace, if you have pictures on your phone, the women that I have worked with over the years love it.

Last, but not least when working with women, and this is real counterculture, but shoot for the work friend zone. Why do I say this? While some of the women at work are going to be going out together, it's going to be a rare; i.e. *every third blue moon* and *only when Saturn's aligned with Venus* day, that you will be invited...anywhere. The only exception may be the workplace picnic or workplace event. If they do have a workplace picnic or get-together, it would definitely be in your best interest to go. It would be in your best interest not to go to anything else with them, but a workplace get-together.

Chapter Four:

Sexual Discrimination, Be Prepared; It Will Happen

I could make this the longest chapter in this guide. I've been through literally every kind of sexual harassment / discrimination there is. These range from being cut down for being a white bald man (I must be a Nazi, don't you know), to having a nurse corner me in the locker room to show me her boob job (then being brought into the nurse manager's office and told not to make a big deal of this because they would hate to have to let me go). I have been harassed for a week to shave my *huevos*, and the list goes on.

So, here are a couple of rules that I've come up with to keep me safe:

First, if at all possible, keep an arms length from any and all women. I know this won't be possible all the time. Ergo, code blues on the floor, to tramas in the E.R., to being beside a patient. In those situations, be very mindful of your surroundings, and make sure you know where all the women in the room are. If you accidentally brush up against a woman, IMMEDIATELY apologize every single time. There was once a code blue, during which I accidentally brushed a womans boob. I apologized at least four times (I was terrified).

Secondly, never be alone with a woman. Use the buddy system, and that's including patients. I know you're a man, and I've also been cut down to for needing help with patients. In this day and age people are lawsuit-happy. It's rare, but if you're alone with a woman, she may make something up for attention. She could do so for money, as well, or perhaps for both. There was one time I had to do an EKG on a female, and I had to lift one of her breasts to put the electrodes on her. After I was done she turned me into the nurse manager and patient advocate for inappropriately touching her. So heed my warning: *NEVER be alone with a woman at work.*

Chapter Five:

So You Fell in Love

It was 1992, and I was working at my local nursing home. The unit I was working on had a shared breakroom with the medicare unit. One day I saw this woman walk into the breakroom, and she was all of 4'11". She had blonde hair pulled back into braids, and huge glasses. They were half the size of her little face, and she was wearing an old-time nurse's dress, and the vintage shoes.

All of the sudden, I was like *Wow this girl is alternative, I've got to meet her*. (Come to find out she got the dress and shoes at the thrift store, and the big ol' glasses for free. She wasn't *trying* to be alternative, she was naturally alternative.) So, I went to break early, and said, "Hi, my name is Chad," and shook her hand. I didn't ask her out for a long time. We just remained work friends, until we started hanging out with the same group of friends. We would all go out for dinner or coffee...lots of coffee. I really wasn't a coffee drinker at the time, and now I can't make it through the day without it.

One night, all of us were at our favorite coffee shop, which was Java Gaya, and the table I was sitting at had a bad leg. I spilled my hot coffee in my lap, and *oh it burned*. I was in so much pain that I forgot where I was. I went to the fancy water fountain in the middle of the place and started splashing water on myself. So, when I came back to myself, I realized that she was gone. (I found out later that she had to run to the bathroom because she was laughing so hard.)

Well, anyway, I decided to gather what little dignity I had left, and head to my car. Then, all of the sudden, I saw her running up to me. She said, "Hey, where are you going?" To make a long story shorter, she said goodbye to her friends, and we took off together. That's when I knew I was interested in her and she might be interested in me. Now, not being the type to turn my back on love, I chose to *approach with caution*, to *take it slow*, to *get to know and trust her first*, before jumping into a serious relationship with her. That made a huge difference for us both.

So, if you find yourself falling in love with someone at work, my advice is: *Relax, take a breath, take it easy, slowly go into this thing, see what type of person she is first.* Is she going to love you for always, or throw you under the bus at the first sign of trouble?

The thought of which takes me to a funny story of a husband/wife nurse duo. They rarely, if ever, worked together. This was until one night, when there was a call in, and he got sent to her unit. Now, it was a busy night. She came up to him and asked for help with something. I can't remember what the *something* was for, but he was swamped and said "I really can't". Oh man, the *fire* in her eyes said, *You better get over here and help me.* He went from swamped to drowning that night. He was taking care of his patients and helping with hers. I felt so bad for him.

Summary:

So, the moral of the story is: When you're a man working in a predominantly female workplace, there are a lot of pros and cons. The pros for me were: *I learned a ton.* Some things a man doesn't need to know, like: *The difference between a pad and a tampon* or *just because the shoes and the dress are the same color doesn't mean they match* or *women's boobs aren't symmetrical ones usually larger/smaller than the other and bras are symmetrical so basically no bra actually fits right.*

Some of what I learned was very useful in my marriage. For example, I learned what a woman will actually respond positively to, like: *Doing the dishes, while laughing and having fun; at the same time.* I learned that, when a woman comes to you venting about this or that, she's not looking for answers. She just wants to vent and have someone listen, and you don't have to have any answers. You just need to listen. That little golden nugget of info was so freeing for me.

Don't say you're helping her out around the house, because it's your house, also. So, pick up a duster and vacuum, and don't say anything. (Trust me, she's watching.) Also, compliment her a lot. If you have a woman of any character, she will reciprocate with her own compliment for you. Now, the cons are: *You have to be careful.* Like: *What you or other men may think are funny may not be funny to a woman.* It may be old-fashioned, but I learned these things from my grandpa: *There's a way to talk and act around men,*

A way to talk and act around women, and *A way to talk and act around children.*

~There is a time and a season for everything.

Ecclesiastes 3:1-8~